EXPLORING CAREERS WITHOUT COLLEGE

VOCATIONAL CAREERS IN HEALTH CARE

by Cynthia Kennedy Henzel

BrightPoint Press

San Diego, CA

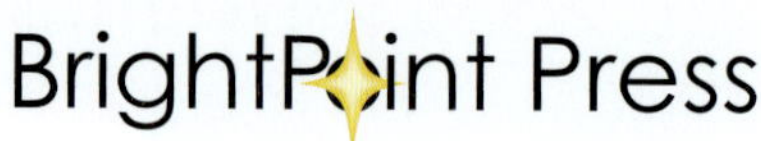

an imprint of ReferencePoint Press, Inc.
Printed in the United States

For more information, contact:
BrightPoint Press
PO Box 27779
San Diego, CA 92198
www.BrightPointPress.com

LIBRARY OF CONGRESS CATALOGING-IN-PUBLICATION DATA

Name: Henzel, Cynthia Kennedy, author.
Title: Vocational careers in health care / by Cynthia Kennedy Henzel.
Description: San Diego, CA: ReferencePoint Press, 2026 | Series: Exploring careers without college | Includes bibliographical references and index. | Audience: Grades 7–9
Identifiers: ISBN 9781678212742 (hardcover) | ISBN 9781678212759 (eBook)
The complete Library of Congress record is available at www.loc.gov.

CONTENTS

THE HEALTH CARE INDUSTRY AT A GLANCE

ANNUAL MEAN WAGE OF SURGICAL TECHNOLOGISTS, 2023

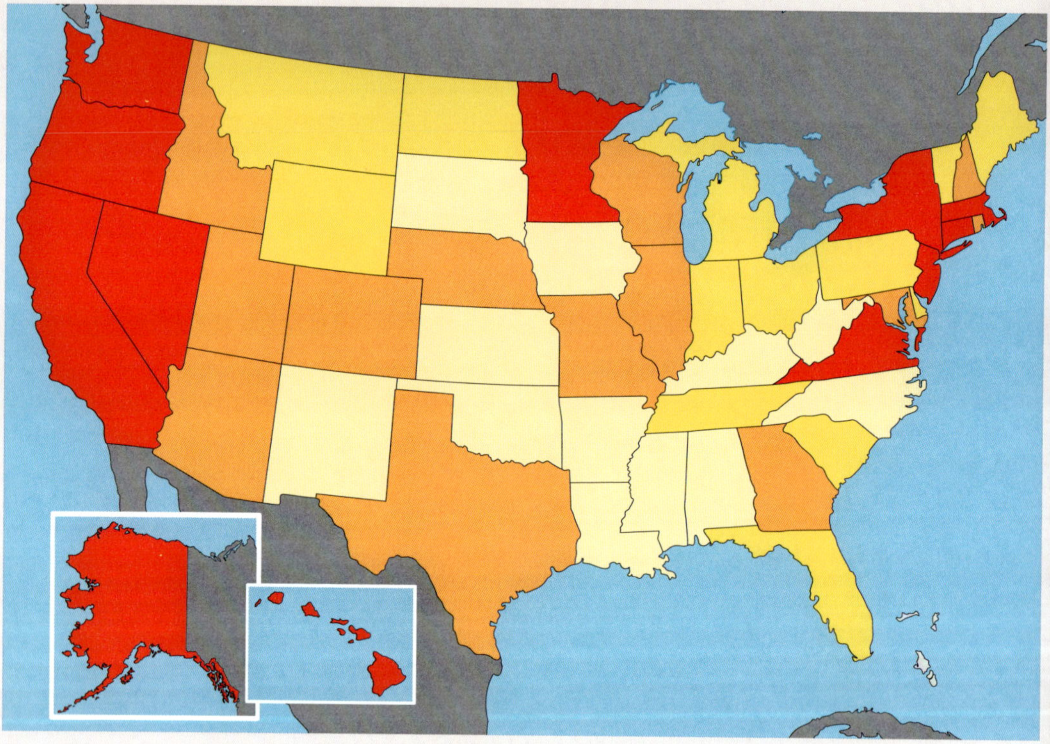

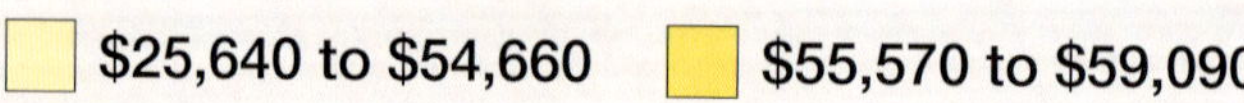

$25,640 to $54,660

$55,570 to $59,090

$59,450 to $66,190

$66,380 to $79,080

Source: "Occupational Employment and Wage Statistics: Surgical Technologists," US Bureau of Labor Statistics, *April 3, 2024, www.bls.gov.*

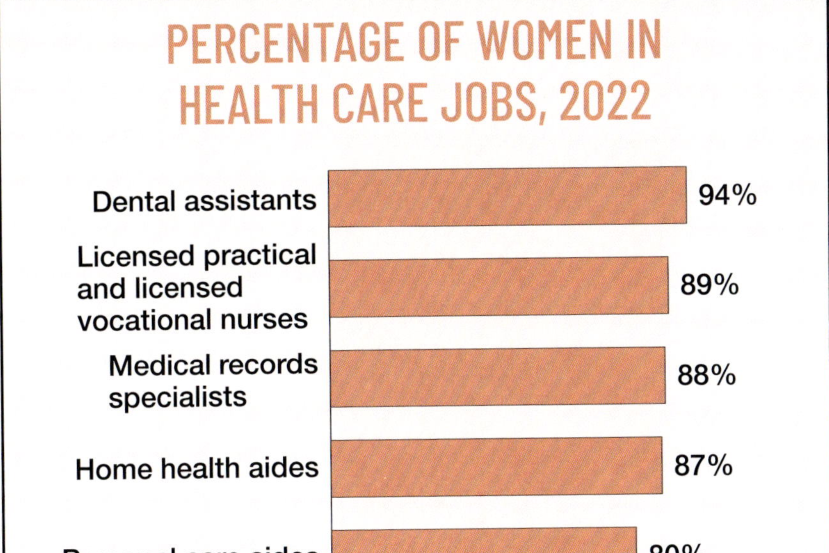

Source: "Spotlight on Statistics: Percent of Women Employees in the 25 Largest Healthcare Occupations, 2022," US Bureau of Labor Statistics, *n.d., www.bls.gov.*

TOP FIVE STATES FOR HOME HEALTH AND PERSONAL CARE AIDE JOBS, 2023

State	Number of Jobs	Annual Wage
California	796,890	$35,220
New York	566,160	$38,280
Texas	312,420	$23,850
Pennsylvania	213,020	$30,580
Massachusetts	113,730	$38,550

Source: "Occupational Employment and Wage Statistics: Home Health and Personal Care Aides," US Bureau of Labor Statistics, *April 3, 2024, www.bls.gov.*

WHAT IS THE HEALTH CARE INDUSTRY?

The man lay on the stretcher. His heart was not beating. He was not breathing. "Start **compressions**," a training officer said. Julia Kim was a new emergency medical technician (EMT). She thought she was ready for this. She had trained on human-sized plastic dolls to do chest compressions. But it was not the same. The life of a person was in her hands.

EMTs are similar to paramedics. However, paramedics have more medical training, which allows them to do advanced procedures.

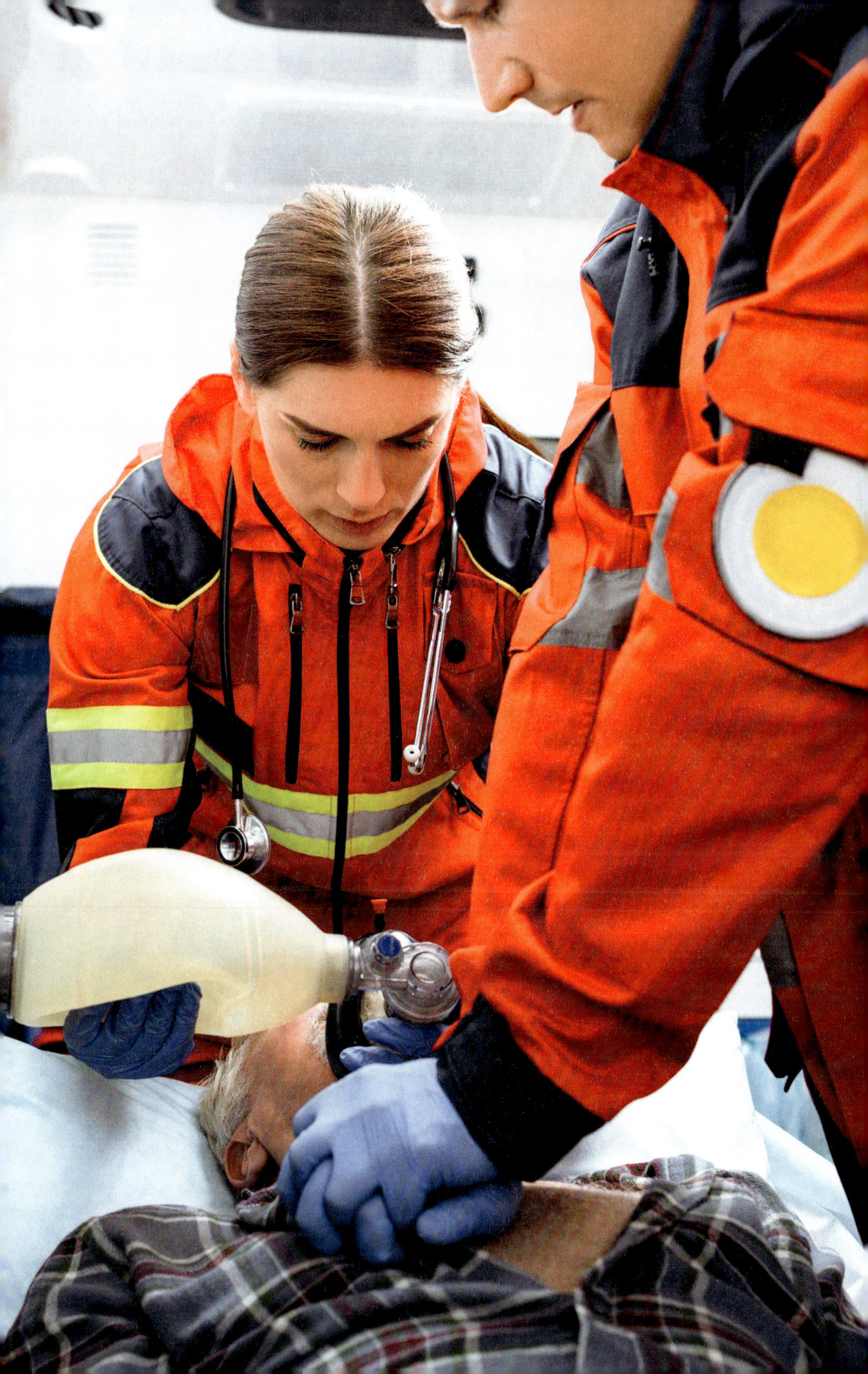

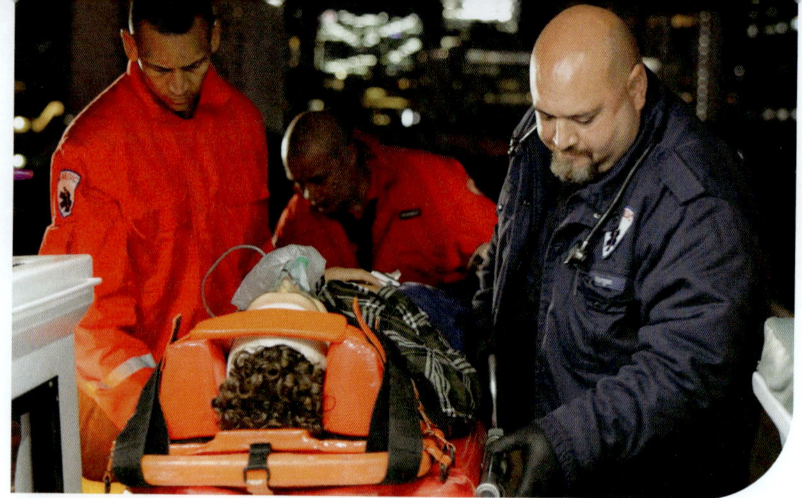

EMTs might have to work nights, weekends, and holidays. They also deal with different kinds of weather, including rain and snow.

Kim pressed up and down on the man's chest for several minutes. Finally, the monitor showed his heart was beating again. Kim and her EMT partner loaded the patient into the ambulance. Her partner drove to the hospital. Kim stayed with the patient. She checked his **vital signs**.

Kim would treat many people as an EMT. She learned to treat everyone with care. And she learned how to remain calm. But Kim would never forget her first patient. That day she learned that medicine was more than skill. It was helping a fellow human.

CAREERS IN HEALTH CARE

The health care industry involves organizations and services that provide medical care. Being an EMT is one of many health care jobs. Some people work in hospitals or doctor's offices. Other health care jobs involve helping doctors during surgeries. Some people might work for dentists.

Health care workers are in high demand. People go into health care for many reasons. The jobs pay well. The variety of opportunities is high. Many people go into health care because they want to help others.

CHAPTER ONE

DENTAL ASSISTANT

Dental assistants work in dentist's offices. They make sure patients are comfortable. Their job includes keeping records. They also schedule appointments. Dental assistants **sterilize** equipment. And they hand supplies to dentists or hygienists when needed.

Many dental assistants take and develop X-rays. Some assistants work in labs. They prepare materials needed to make crowns.

Dental assistants often hold tools called mouth mirrors to help dentists or hygienists see into a patient's mouth.

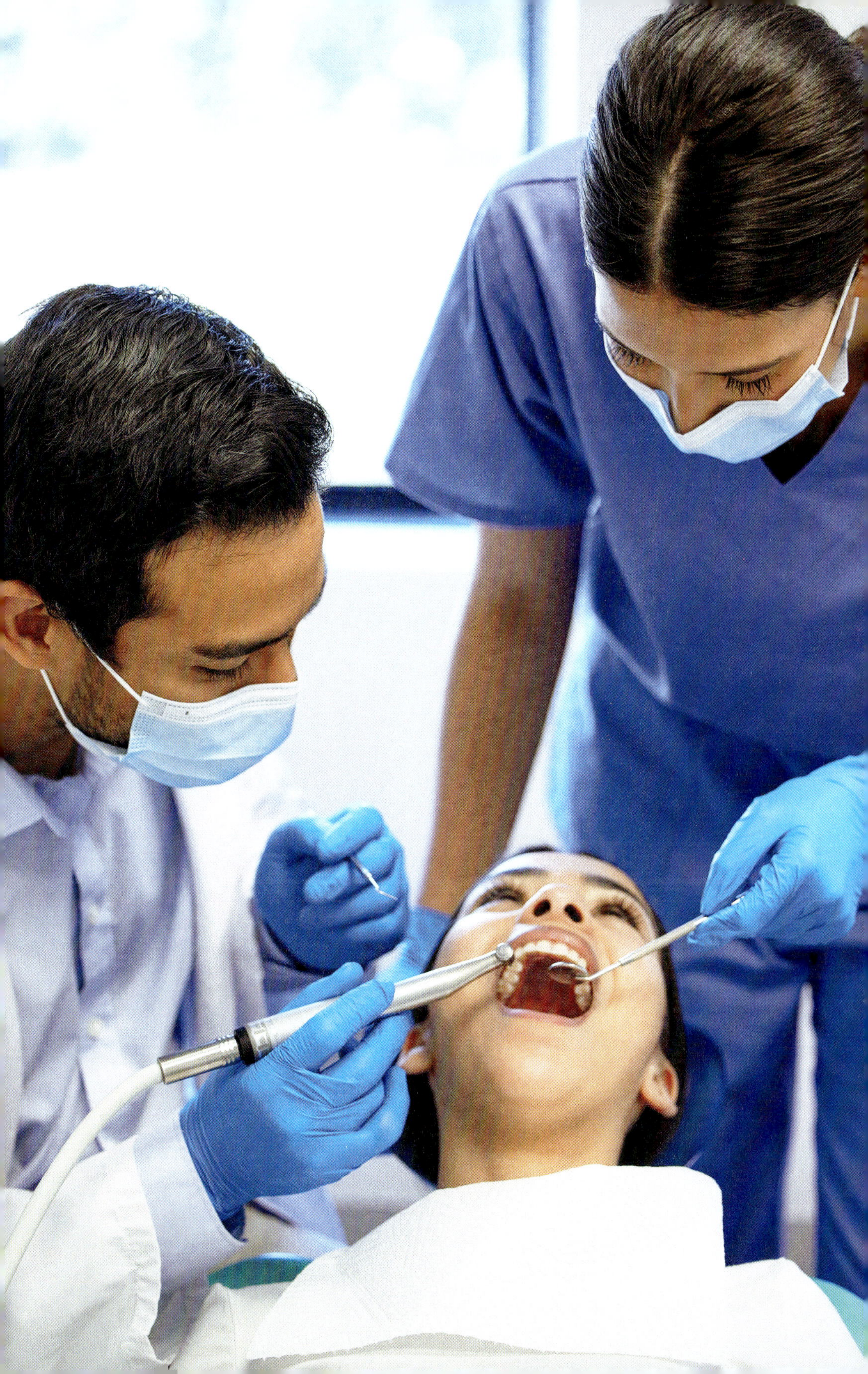

A crown is a cap put over a tooth. This is done to protect the tooth. Dental assistants might take a patient's vital signs. They also explain information to patients. This includes

Dental Assistant

Minimum Education: High school diploma, vocational training (depending on state)

Personal Qualities: Detail oriented, good at working with hands, good social skills

Certification and Licensing: Varies by state. Some states require certification.

Working Conditions: Dental assistants work in offices with dentists and hygienists. They also work with X-ray machines and other dental equipment.

Average Salary: $47,300 (2024)

Number of Jobs: 376,500 (2023)

Future Job Outlook: 8 percent growth expected between 2023 and 2033

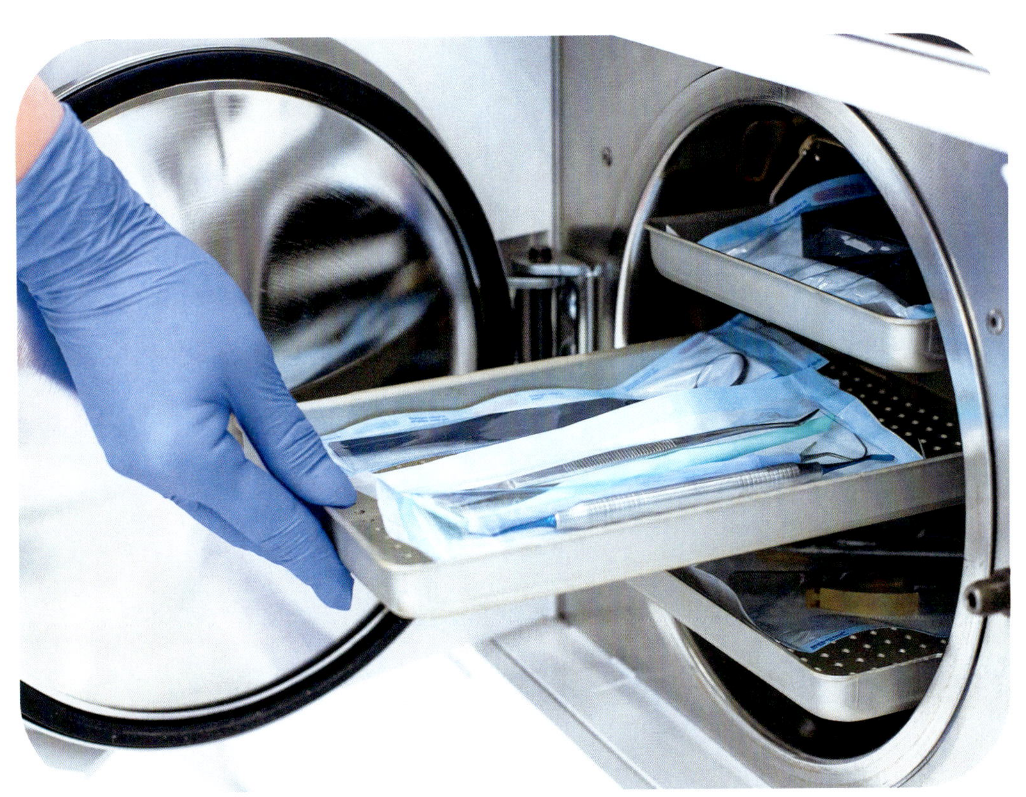

An autoclave is a device that sterilizes medical equipment, such as dental tools.

explaining what will happen during an appointment or procedure.

Connecting with patients is an important part of a dental assistant's job. Many people are scared of going to the dentist. Dental assistants try to make patients feel comfortable. They learn about the patients. They listen to their concerns.

A dental assistant is often the first and last person a patient sees during a visit. Ariel is a children's dental assistant. She says, "I was a very nervous kid at the dentist, so calming my little patients and helping them overcome their fear of the dentist is always a great feeling of accomplishment."[1]

GETTING STARTED

Dental assistants need a high school diploma. They should take science classes. Learning about **anatomy** is important. People should also take biology and chemistry.

Training to become a dental assistant differs by state. Some states require a 1-year program in a vocational school. Students learn about teeth. They learn about the special instruments that dentists and hygienists use. And they get experience by working with someone in the field. The length of the program may be shorter in some states. Programs usually take about 9 months to 1 year.

Other states have no formal educational requirements. They allow on-the-job training. Dental assistant Davina says, "I didn't attend dental assisting school,

Dental Hygienists

Dental hygienists work in a dentist's office. However, their job is different from dental assistants. Hygienists inspect patients for mouth diseases. They clean teeth. Hygienists earn about twice as much as dental assistants. But they require a 3-year degree in dental hygiene.

so my first job in this field was a real eye-opener."[2] New dental assistants can learn **terminology** and instruments by working in a dentist's office.

Dental assistants often need to get certified. Certification proves someone can do a certain job. Dental assistants

Dental assistants should be good at listening to and communicating with people of all ages.

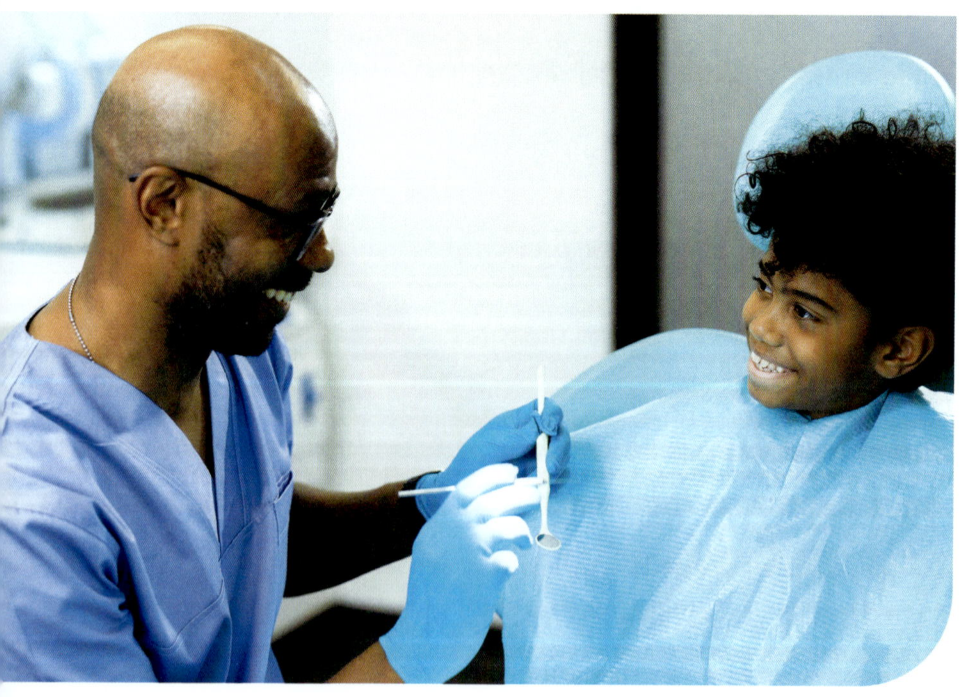

can get a certificate to polish teeth. Other certifications allow assistants to apply sealants and fluoride. These treatments protect teeth from **decay**. The Dental Assisting National Board offers certifications.

ON THE JOB

A dental assistant's job begins before patients arrive. Dental assistants look over the day's schedule. They make sure equipment is sterilized. And they check that supplies are ready. This means making sure items are in the supply room. These items include gauze and cotton balls. Dental assistants also prepare trays for each patient. Trays contain all the tools the dentist or hygienist needs for appointments.

When the first patient arrives, the dental assistant takes them to an exam room. Dental assistants ensure the patient is comfortable. They might ask them about their family or work. Then they explain what will happen during the appointment. They might take X-rays if needed.

When treatment begins, dental assistants hand the dentist or hygienist any tools they need. Assistants adjust the light. They also use a suction hose. This keeps the patient's mouth dry. Other times, dental assistants record what is done as dentists work. These records are used for **insurance**. Or they are used for further treatments.

Once the dentist is done, dental assistants finish the appointment. They talk to the patient about what the dentist did.

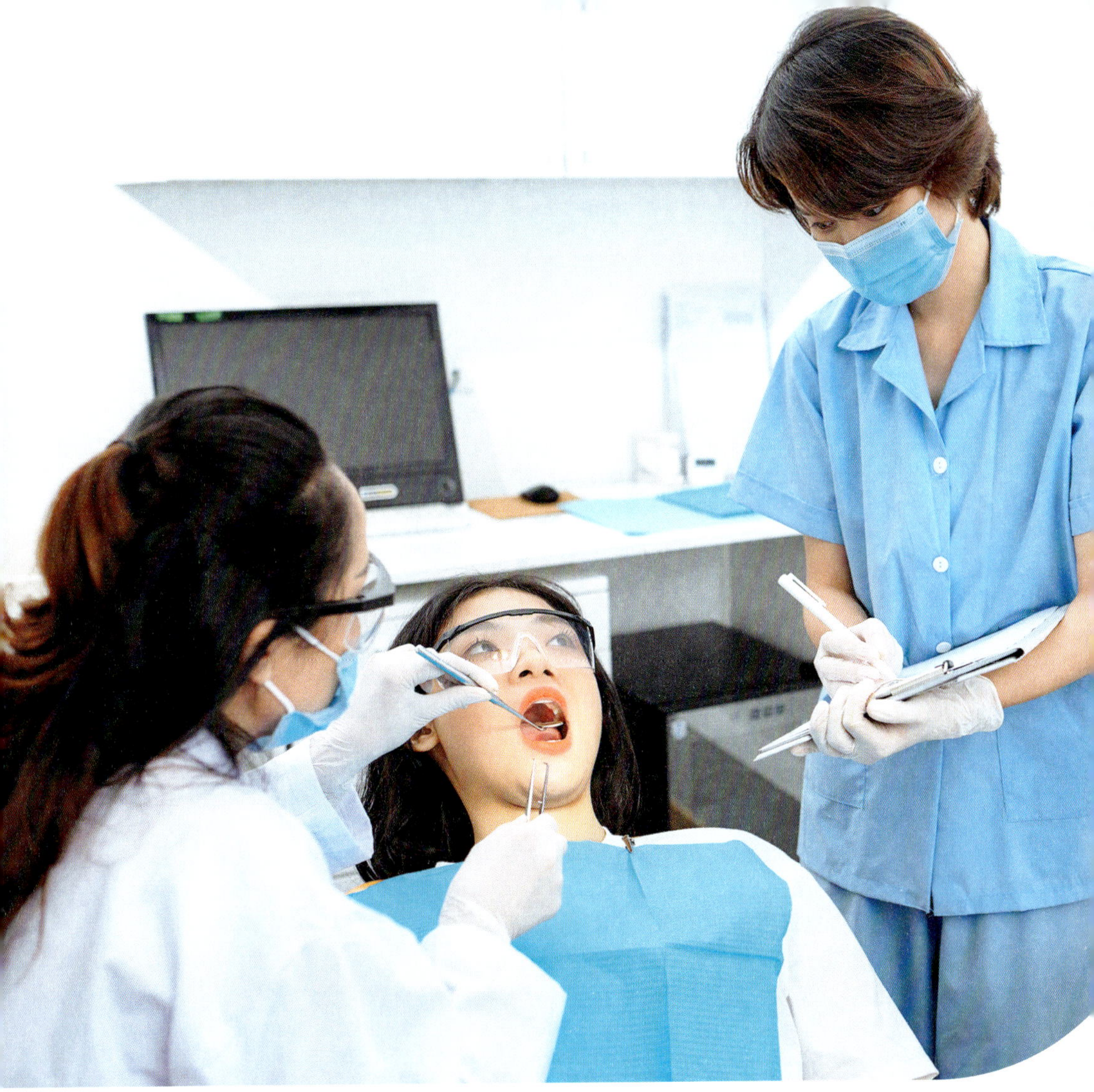

During exams, dental assistants might take notes for dentists and hygienists to help maintain patient records.

They also provide instructions on tooth care. When the patient leaves, assistants prepare the room for the next patient. They clean the room. And they sterilize tools.

Dental assistants may choose different specialties. Cosmetic dentistry focuses on helping people improve their smiles. Some examples include teeth whitening or implants. Pediatric dental assistants work with children. Orthodontic assistants help in the placement and adjustment of braces.

Endodontic assistants work with dentists during surgery. These assistants hand the dentist tools. They also tell the patient what is happening. They may prepare the material to fill a tooth that has a cavity. If dental assistants choose to specialize, they can work toward a certification. Or they can work directly with a specialist to learn the job.

FIND OUT MORE

American Dental Assistants Association
https://adaausa.org
The American Dental Assistants Association (ADAA) is an organization for dental assistants. The ADAA offers online courses, scholarships, and awards for dental assistants.

Dental Assisting National Board
www.danb.org
The Dental Assisting National Board (DANB) provides information about various certifications for dental assistants. The DANB website also has links so people can search for training requirements in different states.

CHAPTER TWO

SURGICAL TECHNOLOGIST

Surgical technologists help surgeons during an operation. They prepare the operating room before a surgery. The room must be sterile. Surgical techs lay out instruments surgeons need. They might prepare the patient for surgery. This is done by cleaning the part of the body that will be operated on. Surgical techs help doctors put on gowns and gloves, too.

Surgical technologists must be familiar with a variety of surgical tools and equipment so they can quickly hand doctors what they need.

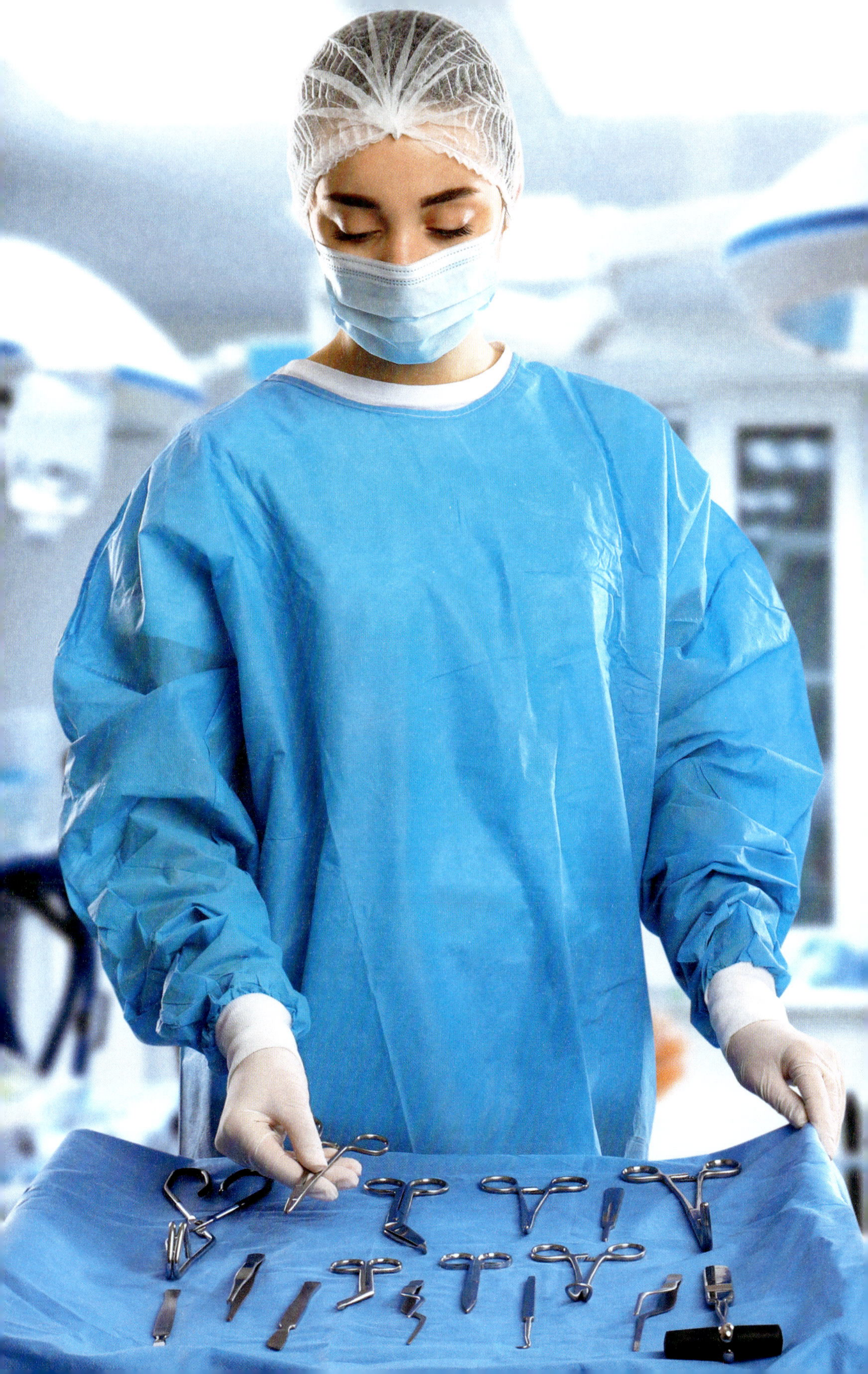

During surgery, techs pass instruments or supplies to surgeons. Techs may help hold organs in place. Doctors might take samples of tissue for testing. Surgical techs

Surgical Technologist

Minimum Education: High school diploma, vocational school

Personal Qualities: Detail oriented, good at working with hands, must work well under pressure

Certification and Licensing: Certification required in most states

Working Conditions: Surgical technologists work in hospitals, and they often spend many hours standing.

Average Salary: $62,480 (2024)

Number of Jobs: 134,000 for surgical technologists and assistants (2023)

Future Job Outlook: 6 percent growth expected between 2023 and 2033

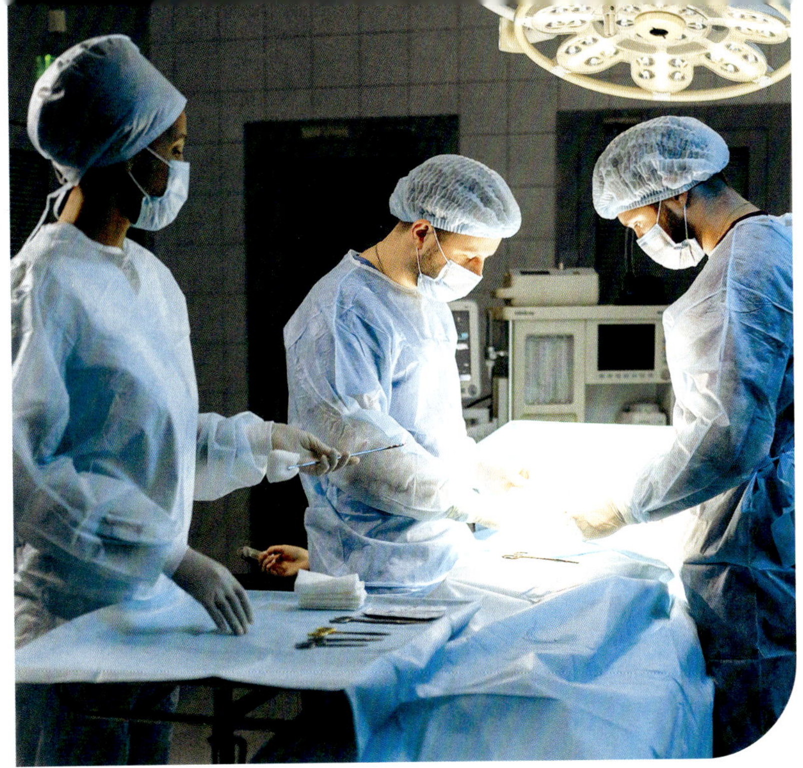

Minor surgeries might take as little as 30 minutes, while some major surgeries can last many hours.

make sure the sample is delivered safely to a lab. After surgery, techs clean the room for the next patient.

GETTING STARTED

Surgical technologists need a high school diploma. They must then do a surgical tech program. This can be done through a vocational school. Students have to

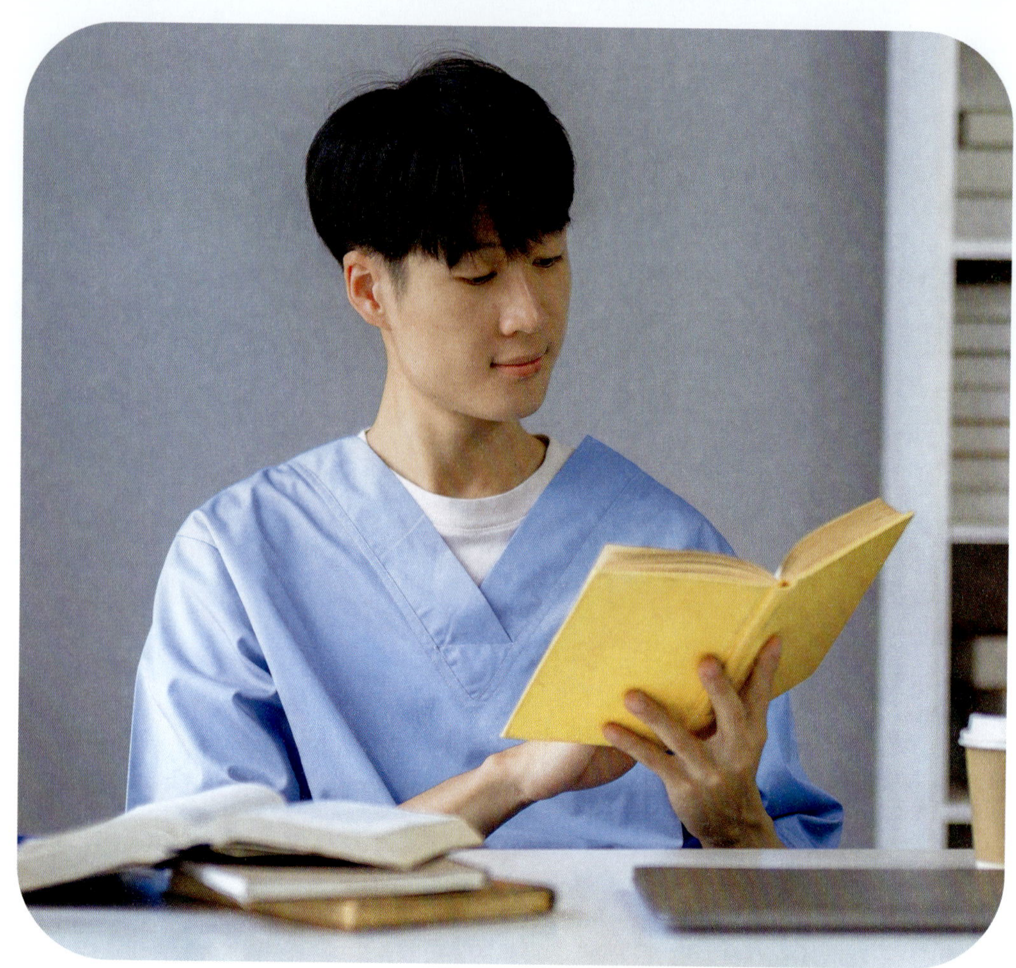

Certified Surgical Technologist and Tech in Surgery are two common certifications for surgical techs. Both require students to take an exam.

take science classes. These include anatomy and microbiology. They also study physiology. Physiology is how the body functions. Vocational programs provide hands-on experience, too.

Many states require surgical techs to be certified. This usually involves taking exams. Surgical tech certification can take as little as 4 months. Some programs can take 1 to 2 years. This is often the case when someone specializes. Certifications are offered by many organizations. One is the National Board of Surgical Technology and Surgical Assisting. Another is the National Center for Competency Testing.

Most techs choose a specialty. This is because different surgeries require certain tools and setup. Some techs work with a doctor who does heart and lung surgeries. Others work with brain doctors. Experienced surgical techs can become surgical assistants. They help doctors more directly during surgery.

ON THE JOB

Most surgical technologists work in hospitals. Some work in dentist's or doctor's offices. The work schedule varies. Hospitals often have 10- or 12-hour workdays. A tech might work 4 days a week. Office jobs usually have 8-hour days.

Many surgeries are scheduled ahead of time. This means techs know when

Surgical Assistants

Surgical assistants are sometimes called first surgical assistants. Both technicians and assistants work in the operating room. But the surgical assistant helps the doctor work on the patient during surgery. They make cuts. They place items to stop bleeding. After surgery, assistants help stitch up patients.

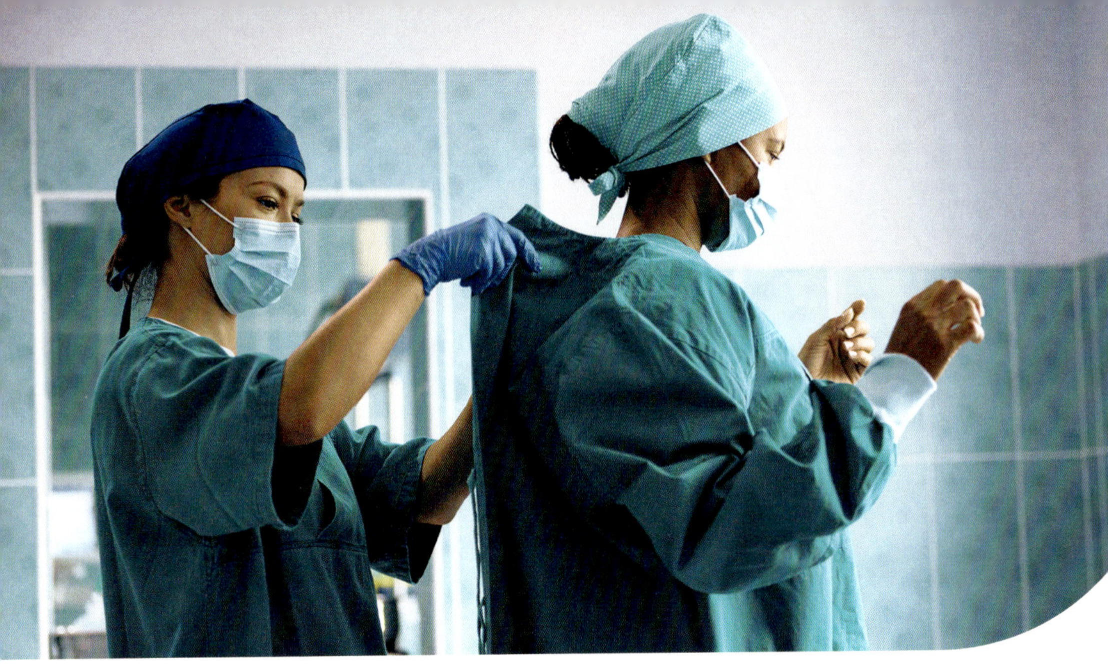

Surgical techs sometimes help surgeons put on sterile gowns and gloves to prevent any diseases from spreading to patients.

they will work. But they may have to work overtime if surgeries take longer than expected. They might also have to work weekends or nights. Sometimes, techs are on call for emergency surgeries. If they are called in, they earn overtime pay.

A surgical tech's workday can start early. When techs arrive, they might change into scrubs. Changing into scrubs keeps patients safe. It prevents bacteria and viruses on regular clothing from getting into the surgical area. Techs change back into regular clothes at the end of the day. This helps prevent the spread of germs. During surgery, techs wear sterile gowns, gloves, caps, and masks.

After surgery, surgical techs make sure medical tools that cannot be used again, such as needles, are properly thrown away.

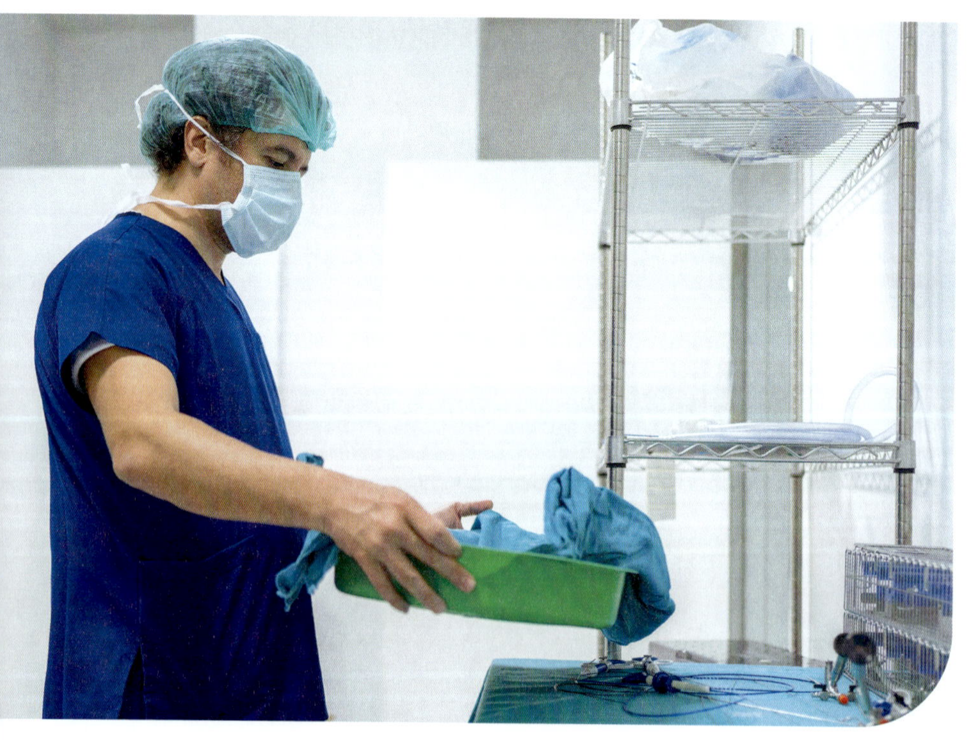

Before an operation, techs prepare the room. Different types of surgeries require various tools. Techs need to know which tools are needed. They also need to know how the surgeon prefers them to be arranged. According to the Mayo Clinic, "The role of the surgical technologist is incredibly important because they ensure a sterile and organized environment."[3]

When everything is ready, the medical team has a time-out. This is a discussion to make sure everyone knows their job. Techs must speak up if they have any concerns.

In the operating room, the patient is given a drug. It puts them into a deep sleep. Then the tech positions the patient so the doctor can operate. Operations can take 30 minutes. Or they can be several hours.

The tech may have to move the patient again during surgery. Techs might have to stand for many hours.

During an operation, techs hand doctors the tools they need. They might also hold organs or tissues in place. As surgery ends, techs count every piece of equipment. "This is such a vital part of the surgery, to make sure that nothing is left in the patient," says surgical tech Jonathan Fillingane.[4]

Working as a surgical tech can be a stressful job. Surgery does not always go as expected. Techs have to respond to whatever happens. But surgical tech Anthony Mareno finds the job rewarding. He says, "You will feel as though you were a part of the team that changed that patient's life forever, and that is because you were!"[5]

FIND OUT MORE

Mayo Clinic College of Medicine and Science
https://college.mayo.edu/academics/explore-health-care-careers/careers-a-z/surgical-technologist
The Mayo Clinic provides a detailed guide about the job of the surgical technologist. It also lists a number of specialties in the field.

National Center for Competency Testing
www.ncctinc.com/certifications/tech-in-surgery-certified
The National Center for Competency Testing (NCCT) is an organization that offers certification for surgical technologists. The NCCT website explains the path to certification from graduating high school to taking the exam.

CHAPTER THREE

MEDICAL RECORDS TECHNICIAN

Medical records technicians (MRTs) manage patient records. They help health organizations run smoothly. MRTs ensure doctors have current information on a patient. This includes the patient's treatment and medical history. MRTs provide information to insurance companies. And they make sure patients can easily access information about their own health care.

MRTs often communicate with patients, doctors, and insurance companies through phone calls and emails.

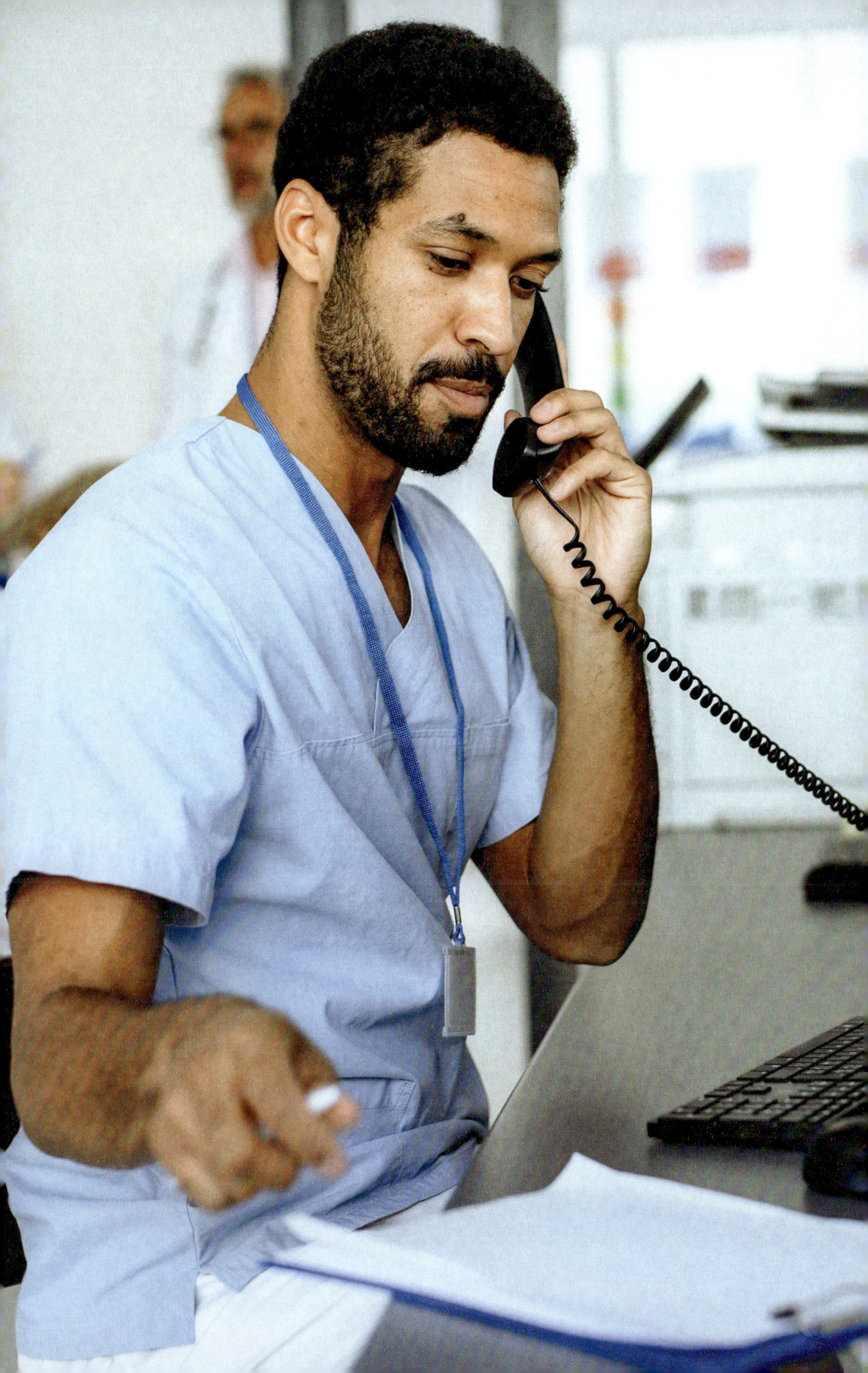

Traci Avis is an MRT. Avis knew she wanted to work in health care. But she did not think she could work with very ill patients. "I'm way too emotional," she said.[6]

Medical Records Technician

Minimum Education: High school diploma, technical school

Personal Qualities: Analytical skills, interpersonal skills, trustworthiness

Certification and Licensing: Certification required for most positions

Working Conditions: Medical records technicians work at computers, either in an office or from home. Most work during the weekdays, although some might work on nights and weekends.

Average Salary: $50,250 (2024)

Number of Jobs: 191,500 (2023)

Future Job Outlook: 9 percent growth expected between 2023 and 2033

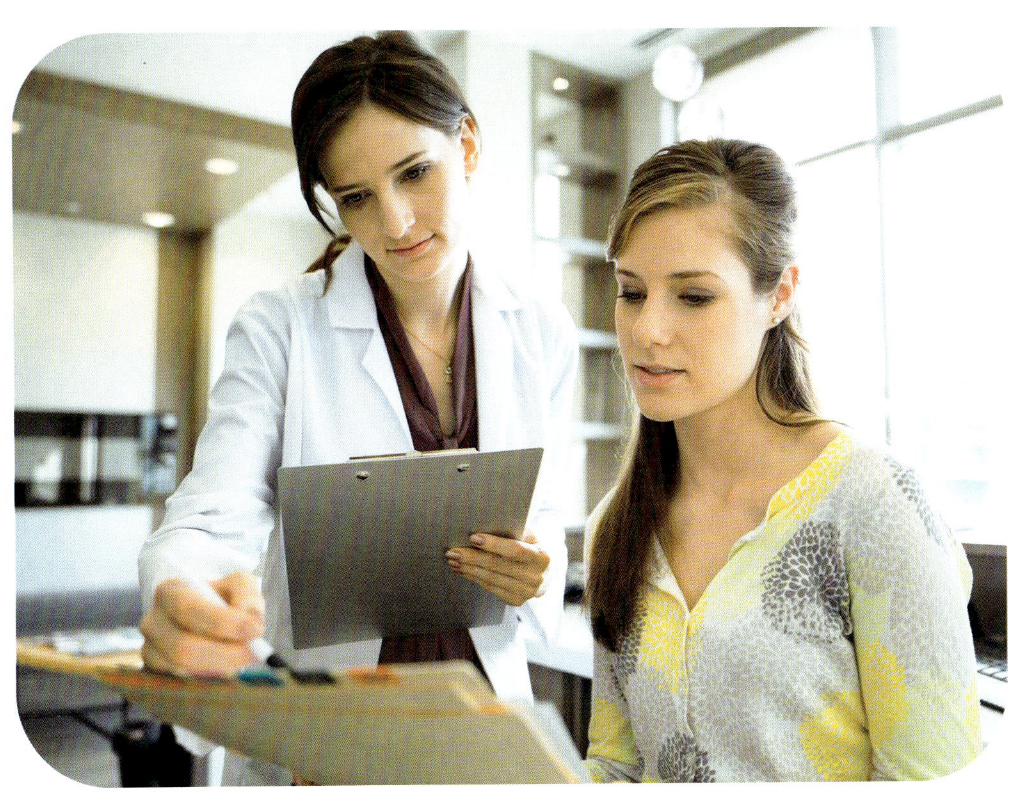

Confirming patient procedures and treatments is an important part of an MRT's job.

Being an MRT allowed Avis to work in the field without the stress of patient care.

MRTs work with electronic health records. These contain results from doctor's appointments or hospital stays. Records are kept online. This allows medical professionals to quickly access information about a patient's medical care.

MRTs also add new appointments or lab tests. This information is used to bill the insurance and patient. MRTs carefully check records for accuracy. A simple error can delay patient treatment. They also make sure patient records are kept private. MRTs check that anyone who wants access to records has the patient's permission.

GETTING STARTED

MRTs need a high school diploma. They need to develop computer skills. Science classes are useful, too. These include biology and anatomy. Science classes can help MRTs learn about the human body.

After high school, most MRTs get certified. They might take classes at a technical school. MRTs learn medical terms.

This helps them understand notes written by doctors. They must enter those notes into the patient's record. MRTs also learn about special coding used to record patient data. These codes let everyone in the health care system understand a patient's **diagnosis** and treatment plan.

Specialists in medical records may work in a particular area of medical care. For example, cancer registrars work only

MRTs help convert paper records to digital so health care providers and insurance companies have easier access to them.

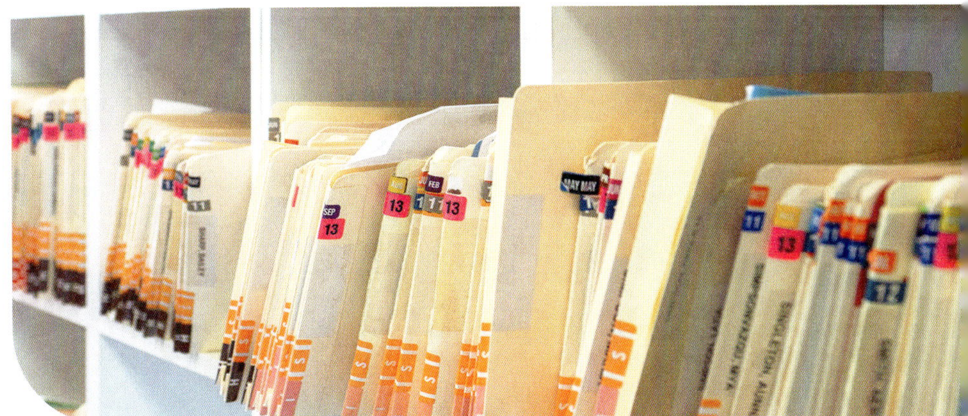

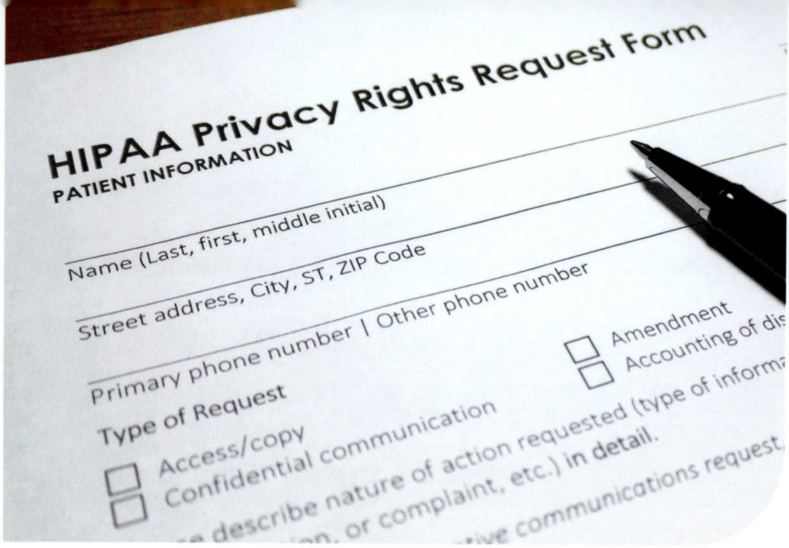

The Health Insurance Portability and Accountability Act was established on August 21, 1996.

with cancer patients. Registrars keep track of official records. They assign codes. That data goes to databases across the United States. It is used by those who research cancer treatments and recovery.

MRTs need analytical skills. They must understand medical records to assign a diagnosis code. They must be precise in recording and checking data. MRTs need to be trustworthy. The Health Insurance Portability and Accountability Act (HIPAA) protects patient privacy. HIPAA rules limit who can access patient data. The MRT ensures these rules are followed. This keeps patient information private.

ON THE JOB

Most MRTs work in a hospital. Some work in a doctor's office. Others work for nursing homes or insurance companies. MRTs usually work 8 hours during the weekdays.

Medical Coding Specialists

Medical coding specialists assign codes for medical systems. Codes are used when working with companies and agencies that pay for health care. Coders review medical charts. They determine which codes are best for a certain diagnosis. Medical coders use the ICD-10. This is the tenth revision of the International Classification of Diseases.

But those who work in hospitals might work weekends or evenings. Since MRTs use computers, some can work from home.

MRTs start the day by checking their email. Responding to records requests quickly is important. A delay in providing information means the patient has to wait for treatment. A doctor may need information about past treatment. Or the billing department may need details about an insurance issue.

After requests are filled, the MRT opens the electronic health records system. This software stores patient data. The medical records have information on previous symptoms and diagnoses. MRTs update that data. They add doctors' notes. They check that known allergies are recorded. And they add any new prescriptions.

Throughout the day, MRTs get new requests for records. They work quickly with nurses, doctors, and other staff to find the needed information. A patient may request

Staying organized and being detail oriented are important skills for MRTs. This ensures patients' records and results are correctly labeled and filed.

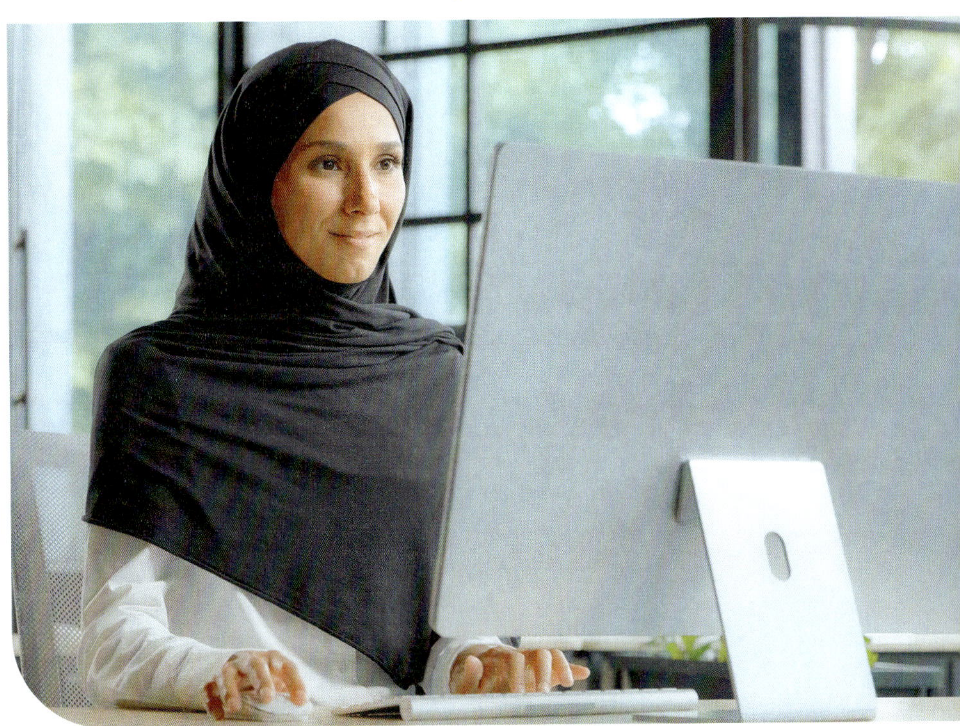

a copy of their records. A doctor might need a file before continuing treatment. MRTs must organize these requests. Then those requests must be sent in a timely manner.

MRTs also create files for new patients. Data on a patient's medical history is recorded. MRTs confirm insurance information. When a patient leaves a hospital or ends treatment, MRTs make sure their record is up to date. Kathy Nussbaum works with medical records. She says:

> *I love working as a health information professional because I feel like we are the bridge between the hospitals and the completion of a patient's treatment with us.*[7]

FIND OUT MORE

HealthJob
www.healthjob.org/guide/how-to-become-a-medical-records-technician
HealthJob offers a detailed guide to becoming a medical records technician. The site also offers some suggestions for online training.

National Healthcareer Association
www.nhanow.com/certification/nha-certifications/certified-electronic-health-records-specialist-(cehrs)
The National Healthcareer Association (NHA) provides information on training to become a health records technician. The NHA also has information on taking the exam for certification.

CHAPTER FOUR

HOME HEALTH AIDE

A home health aide (HHA) helps people when they are ill or disabled. They take care of people in their homes. Aides help patients with their medical care. They make sure patients take medication. They take vital signs. And they change bandages. An HHA helps patients get to doctor's appointments. They also keep records about how a patient is doing.

Home health aides need to have good physical strength to do tasks such as lifting patients from beds or wheelchairs and helping patients stand.

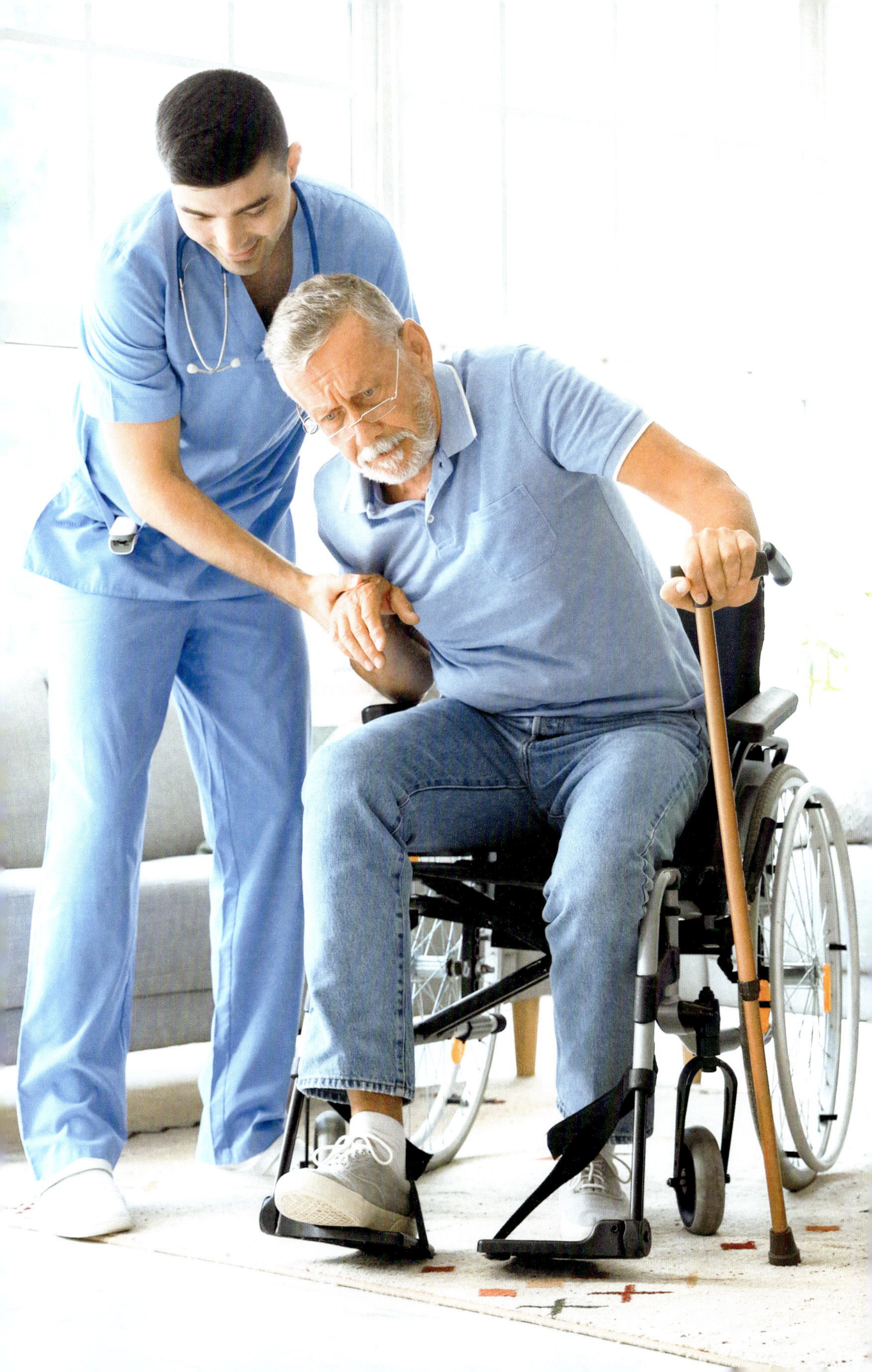

HHAs assist with activities people do every day. This includes bathing or getting dressed. Other patients need help with household chores, such as washing dishes.

Home Health Aide

Minimum Education: High school diploma, on-the-job training

Personal Qualities: Caring about others, kindness, physical strength, trustworthiness

Certification and Licensing: Licensing and certification required in some states

Working Conditions: Home health aides usually work in a patient's home. Aides may have to lift people or heavy objects and deal with difficult patients.

Average Salary: $34,900 (2024)

Number of Jobs: 3,961,900 for home health aides and personal care aides (2023)

Future Job Outlook: 21 percent growth expected between 2023 and 2033

Aides keep patients safe at home. They also help patients stay a part of their community. They might help patients take walks outside, too.

Aides pay attention to details. They carefully follow instructions from doctors or nurses. An HHA must be caring. Patients sometimes have extreme pain or distress. Aides must be trustworthy. People depend on them.

GETTING STARTED

Most aides are required to have high school diplomas. Students then need training. The US government requires HHAs to have at least 75 hours of training. This is needed to work for agencies that get government funds.

Some states require HHAs to get certified or licensed. Many vocational schools offer home health aide certifications. One common HHA requirement is cardiopulmonary resuscitation (CPR) certification. CPR is a medical technique. It is used if a person's heart stops beating.

During CPR training, people practice on adult and child dolls to learn how to properly perform the technique.

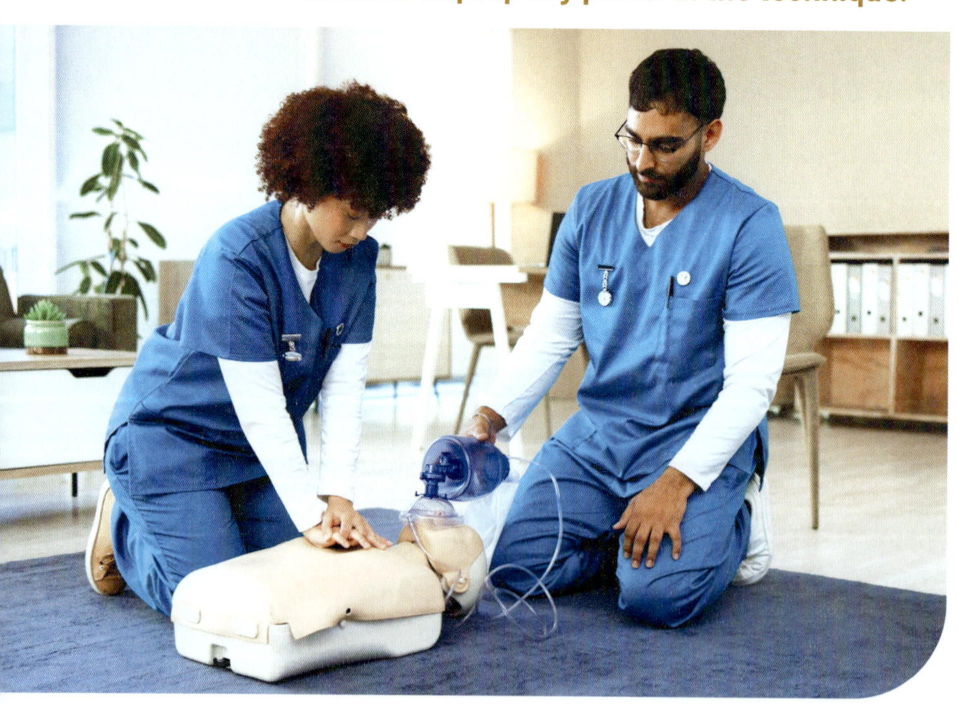

Or it is used when someone stops breathing. Aides may also need to certify in basic life support (BLS). BLS is a set of emergency procedures to do in a life-threatening event. Most companies that hire HHAs provide short on-the-job training.

Some employers require aides to have a background check. Background checks make sure a person is telling the truth about who they are. They also confirm past employment. And they search for criminal records.

HHAs can provide different services depending on the state. Some can check a patient's temperature and pulse. They might help people do exercises prescribed by doctors. Sometimes, they help with braces or artificial limbs. Others may be trained to help with medical equipment. This includes ventilators. These are machines that help a patient breathe.

ON THE JOB

Most HHAs work in a patient's home. They may work with one patient. Or they may work with several patients at different homes. Others work in assisted living.

Travel Trainer

Travel trainers help older adults and people with disabilities use public transportation. They work with people one-on-one. Trainers help plan shopping trips or visits to doctors. They teach people how to use the bus system. And they show people what to do if they get lost. Skills for travel trainers include being organized and enjoying helping people.

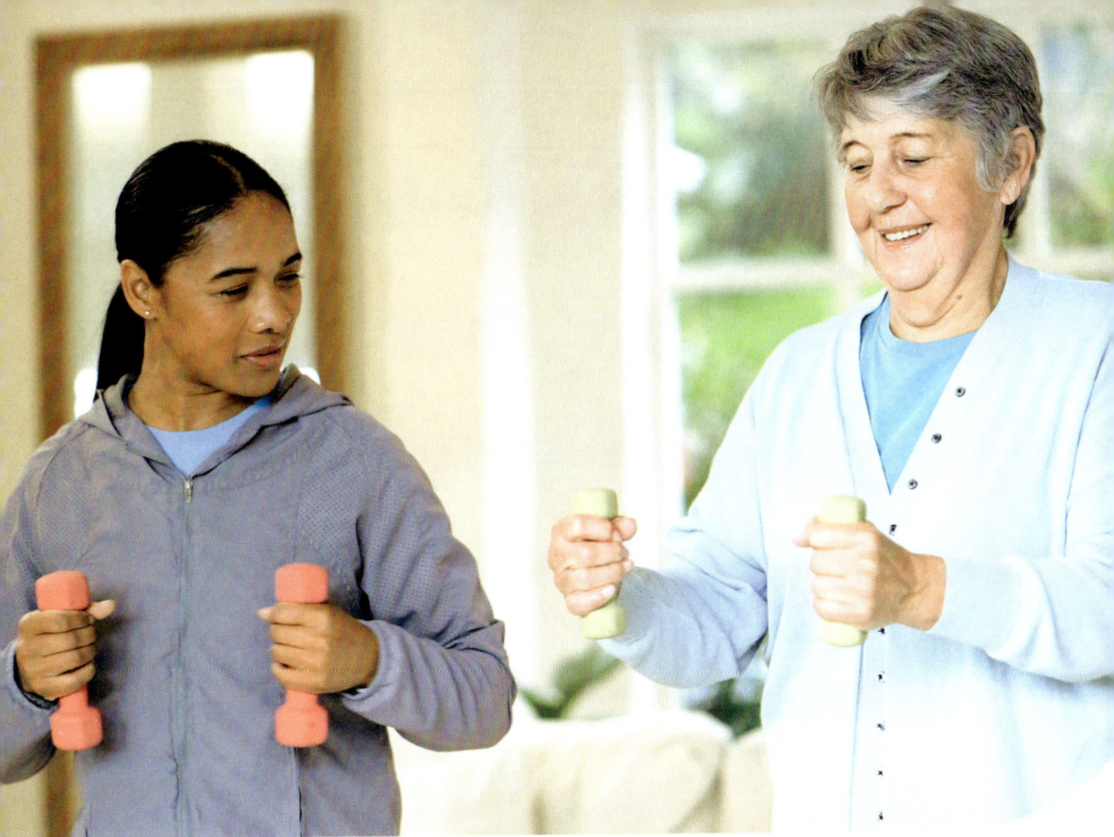

Home health aides ensure patients do their prescribed exercises safely and correctly.

These communities provide services to people who cannot safely live alone.

At the beginning of the day, HHAs check the schedule. Some patients need only a short visit every day. Aides may visit for an hour in the morning. What they do depends on the patient's needs. They might help someone dress. Or they change a bandage.

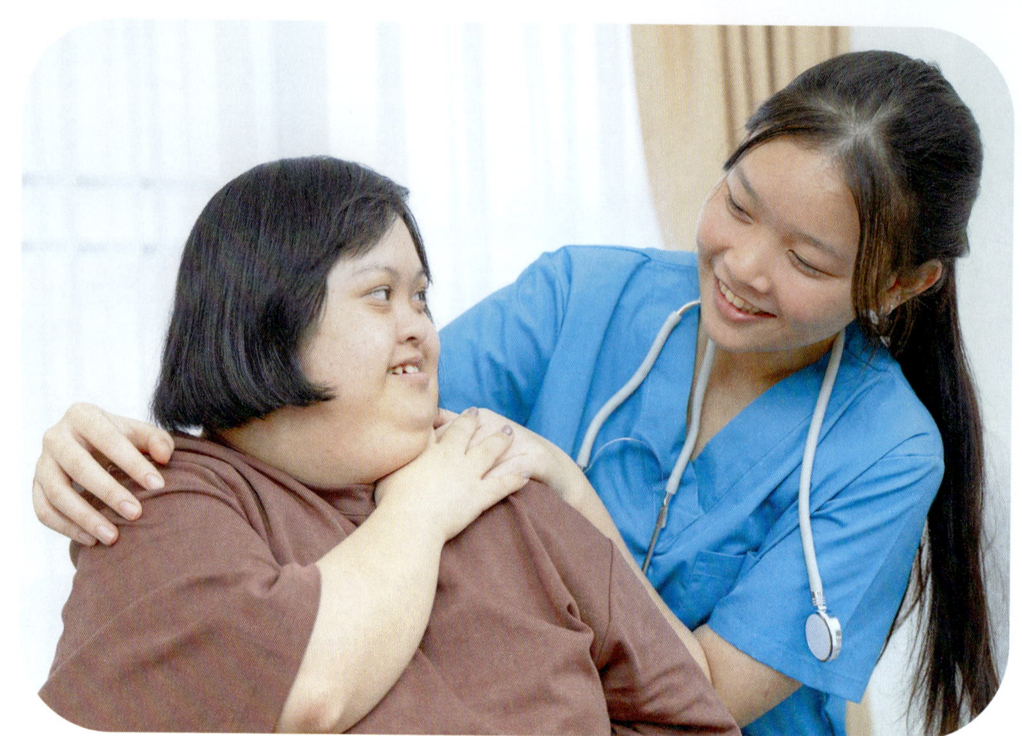

Home health aides provide support so patients with illnesses and disabilities can maintain their independence.

HHAs give medication. They may feed a patient. Other times, aides help patients bathe or use the toilet. They may assist when the patient moves into a wheelchair or vehicle.

HHAs then go to the next patient's home. If a patient is recovering from an accident, they might need only short-term care.

Other patients need more time with aides. Some may need care for the rest of their lives.

Another important part of an HHA's job is caring for the patient's mental health. An aide may be the only person a patient sees during a day. They might talk with the patient. Sometimes, they do activities with the patient. An aide is an important part of the medical team. But they are also an important part of their patient's daily life.

Aides keep detailed records of a patient's problems. They also keep track of a patient's progress. They report this information to a doctor or nurse. Indira Ortiz is an HHA. She states, "The visit isn't complete until the paperwork is in!"[8] Before another visit, the HHA may talk to a team member. They might discuss changes to what they will do on their next visit.

Being an HHA can be stressful. Working in someone's home is not like working in a hospital. It is not a sterile workplace. Aides must be careful to wear gloves and masks. These keep the patient and the aide safe. Patients who have mental health problems may display violent behavior. Aides must stay calm in these situations.

However, being an HHA can be a rewarding job. Kenzie Hawkins is an aide. She says, "I enjoy getting to know new people, hearing their stories, learning about their lives, and how grateful they are for the service we provide."[9]

FIND OUT MORE

National Alliance for Care at Home
https://allianceforcareathome.org
The National Alliance for Care at Home is an organization that helps educate and support people working in home health care. The site offers resources along with information on events and certifications for aides.

PHI
www.phinational.org/advocacy/home-health-aide-training-requirements-state-2016
PHI is a nonprofit organization that works to protect health care in the United States. Its website features a map so people can find training requirements for home health aides by state.

OTHER JOBS IN THE HEALTH CARE INDUSTRY

Optician

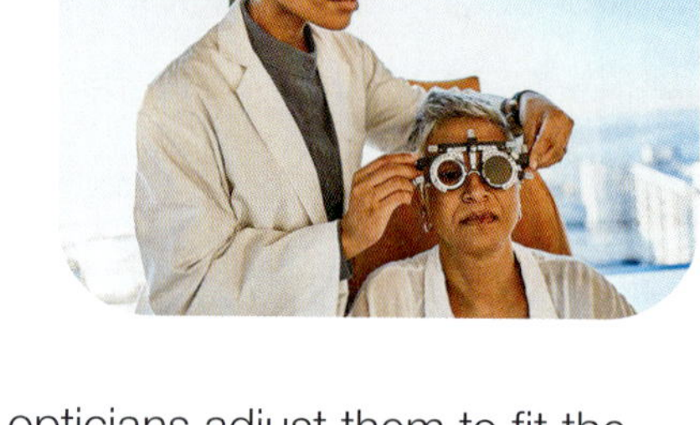

Opticians fit customers for eyeglasses or contact lenses. They measure a customer's face and the distance between their pupils. Then they help customers select frames or contacts. Opticians create work orders at the place that makes lenses and frames. When glasses arrive, opticians adjust them to fit the customer. Or they help customers insert or remove contact lenses. They also show people how to care for eyewear.

Phlebotomist

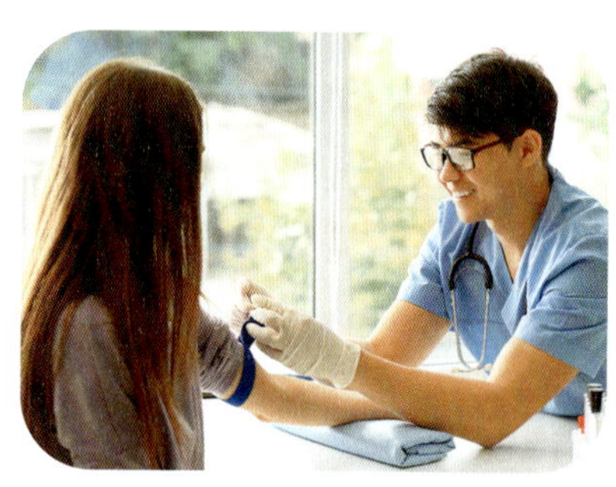

Phlebotomists draw blood from patients or blood donors. Drawing blood requires inserting a needle into a vein. The blood then flows into a tube. Phlebotomists may draw blood for medical tests. Or they may do it for research. During blood drives, phlebotomists draw blood from people who are giving blood to help others. Phlebotomists must be patient with people who are scared of needles. They must also label containers correctly and keep careful records.

Licensed Practical Nurse

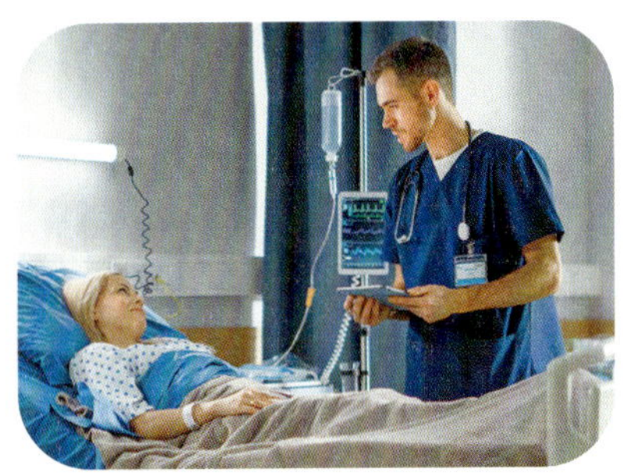

Licensed practical nurses (LPNs) provide basic care to patients. They take vital signs. They care for and bandage wounds. LPNs help patients understand their treatment plan. Or they may help patients dress, bathe, or eat. LPNs are supervised by doctors and nurses. In some states, they may give medication or start intravenous (IV) drips. Other states require these duties to be performed by a licensed vocational nurse.

Emergency Medical Technician

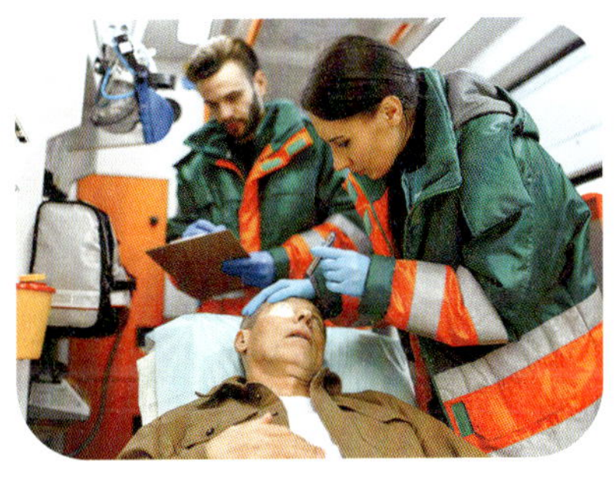

Emergency medical technicians (EMTs) respond to health emergencies, such as heart attacks or car accidents. They assess injuries or illnesses. Then they provide emergency care, such as stopping bleeding or doing CPR. EMTs prepare patients to ride in an ambulance. Then they transport the patient to a hospital for further treatment. EMTs sometimes work with paramedics. Paramedics require more training and are allowed to do more medical procedures.

GLOSSARY

anatomy

the study of the parts of the human body

compressions

a medical technique that involves pushing up and down on a person's chest to try to start their heart

decay

rot caused by bacteria

diagnosis

the identification of a disease using signs and symptoms

insurance

an arrangement in which a person pays a company to help pay in the event of an emergency, accident, or sickness

sterilize

to remove bacteria or other organisms

terminology

specific words used in a particular field

vital signs

measurements of the body's basic functions, including temperature, heart rate, and breathing rate

SOURCE NOTES

CHAPTER ONE: DENTAL ASSISTANT

1. Quoted in "4 Joys of Being a Pediatric Dental Assistant," *Dental Assisting National Board*, August 17, 2023. www.danb.org.

2. Davina A., "How Do You Like Being a Dental Assistant? Davina's Answer," *CareerVillage.org*, June 16, 2023. www.careervillage.org.

CHAPTER TWO: SURGICAL TECHNOLOGIST

3. "Surgical Technologist," *Mayo Clinic*, n.d. https://college.mayo.edu.

4. Quoted in Carrie Mesrobian, "Surgical Technologist Duties: A Day in the Life," *Rasmussen University*, May 9, 2022. www.rasmussen.edu.

5. Quoted in Mesrobian, "Surgical Technologist Duties: A Day in the Life."

CHAPTER THREE: MEDICAL RECORDS TECHNICIAN

6. Quoted in Emily H. Bratcher, "Medical Records Technician," *US News and World Report*, n.d. https://money.usnews.com.

7. Quoted in "7 Reasons Why We Love Being a Health Information Professional," *Northwell Health*, n.d. https://jobs.northwell.edu.

CHAPTER FOUR: HOME HEALTH AIDE

8. Indira Ortiz, "A Day in the Life of a Home Health Aide/Health Coach," *National Library of Medicine*, June 2016. https://pmc.ncbi.nlm.nih.gov.

9. Quoted in Angela Petersen, "A Day in the Life of a Home Care Aide," *Snyder Village*, June 17, 2022. www.snydervillage.com.

INDEX

IMAGE CREDITS

Cover: © Max Acronym/Shutterstock Images
4: Red Line Editorial
5: Red Line Editorial
7: © LightField Studios/Shutterstock Images
8: © PeopleImages.com-Yuri A./Shutterstock Images
11: © PeopleImages.com-Yuri A./Shutterstock Images
13: © Gorynvd/Shutterstock Images
16: © RgStudio/iStockphoto
19: © Dragon Images/Shutterstock Images
23: © New Africa/Shutterstock Images
25: © Dikushin Dmitry/Shutterstock Images
26: © Wichayada Suwanachun/Shutterstock Images
29: © Drazen Zigic/Shutterstock Images
30: © AquaArts Studio/iStockphoto
35: © Halfpoint/iStockphoto
37: © Hero Images Inc/Shutterstock Images
39: © stphillips/iStockphoto
40: © Hailshadow/iStockphoto
43: © Maya Lab/Shutterstock Images
47: © Pixel-Shot/Shutterstock Images
50: © PeopleImages.com-Yuri A./Shutterstock Images
53: © PeopleImages.com-Yuri A./Shutterstock Images
54: © Attasit Saentep/Shutterstock Images
58 (top): © PeopleImages.com-Yuri A./Shutterstock Images
58 (bottom): © Pixel-Shot/Shutterstock Images
59 (top): © Gorodenkoff/Shutterstock Images
59 (bottom): © Orion Production/Shutterstock Images

ABOUT THE AUTHOR

Cynthia Kennedy Henzel has degrees in education and geography. She has written more than a hundred books for young people. These include fiction and nonfiction on subjects such as geography, science, culture, and history. She enjoys learning new things and sharing them with others. Henzel is thankful for all the people who work in health care. Their work makes a big difference to people everywhere.